HOLISTIC MEDICINE FOR WOMEN'S HEALTH

Fighting Some Of Her Most Common Ailments

by

SAUCIRON

Holistic Medicine For Women's Health
Fighting Some Of Her Most Common Ailments
By Sauciron

*I would like to dedicate this book to my mother
Mrs. Jean Elizabeth Harvey who helped countless
elderly people even as she became elderly. Her endless
devotion to helping the needy inspires me to this day.*

Contents

Introduction

My goal is to keep you informed of the various ways to attain and retain optimal natural health resulting from the use of vitamin, herbal, and mineral supplements. No drugs will be recommended because they frequently cause serious side effects. I think there's a better way to get healthy and stay healthy. And that better way is by consuming organic foods, vitamin, herbal, and mineral supplements.

Super-bugs are gaining a foothold in our society and we need to address the issue right now. The major offenders are e-Coli, SARS, Salmonella, and Staph Infections. These so called super bugs have spawned at least 40 new antibiotic resistant diseases in the last 25 years and we can expect many more in the near future.

So how did these super bugs get started? Back in the 1940's during World War II, penicillin and other antibiotics saved thousands of lives due to their ability to fight infections and wartime injuries. After the war, doctors began prescribing antibiotics for almost every illness, even the common cold. This created a strange reaction. The more antibiotics a person takes, the quicker an infection will find a new and more devastating way to attack your body. And this new way will be antibiotic resistant.

If you don't take antibiotics on a regular basis, don't think you are not involved in the big picture. If you eat grain fed beef, pork, or chicken you are consuming antibiotics from the meat you eat. Cows, pigs, and chickens are now being raised in large numbers to meet global demands. During this process, some of the animals get sick so they are all fed antibiotic laden feed to keep them from getting sick. When you eat the meat, small quantities of those antibiotics get into your system and over the years they begin to build up making you prone to a potential attack from an antibiotic resistant super-bug.

Enough of all that depressing news, here's some good news. Numerous supplements are classified as natural antibiotics and you can fortify your immune system by taking them on a regular basis.

I invite you to browse the following chapters. You will learn much more about herbs, vitamins, minerals, and how they can keep you healthy without troublesome side effects.

About the Author

Twenty years ago my mother had a series of mini-strokes. I took care of her at home because many years earlier she had asked me not to put her in a nursing home if it was at all possible. Her doctor explained her situation and it went something like this. "Your mother's strokes have caused permanent brain damage. Her brain cells are slowly dying and the cells adjacent to the damaged cells will eventually die also. I'm sorry, but there's nothing we can do for her".

The mainstream medical community had given up on the person most dear to me. So I decided to conduct some extensive research into alternative measures like vitamins, herbs, and minerals. I was determined not to let my mother die without a fight. This is the person who took care of me when I was sick; she deserved the same from me.

I read multitudes of books, newsletters, and reports. I watched educational videos, attended homeopathic trade-shows, and interviewed anyone who would be willing to talk to me. All the time taking extensive notes and documenting my efforts. I fought an endless fight, but I lost my mother. I started too late in her illness.

After a period of mourning and occasional bouts of depression, I decided to take all that valuable information I had accumulated, continue my research, and use it to help others.

If you are a young woman, don't take life for granted. Supplementation now can keep you healthy into your senior years and beyond. If you are an older person, still healthy or with health issues, supplementation can help you in either case. The following pages will feature some of the health issues women face and how to prevent and treat them with the help of dietary supplements and organic foods.

Here's wishing you health, longevity, and a happy high quality of life. Breast Cancer presents a serious threat to women's health but, as you well know, there are numerous other threats like Heart Disease, Lupus, Fibromyalgia and numerous others. Some are life threatening and others make your quality of life extremely poor. If you're looking for a natural approach to women's health issues without those pesky pharmaceutical side effects, go to vitaminandherbalhealth.com.

A Note To The Reader

When we emerge from the safety and sterility of the womb, 98% of us are healthy little people free of all the health hazards waiting for us in this new environment. Forty or so years later, however, that healthy 98% has decreased substantially. Why ? Well it seems as if some of that group picked up some bad habits along the way. Bad habits like smoking, excessive alcohol consumption, drug use both legal and illegal, and numerous other bad habits that are detrimental to their health. And now, years later, you guessed it, they are having health problems.

Other members of that original group who didn't pick up those bad habits are patting each other on the backs and giving congratulatory high fives. That all ended when they got some disturbing news. Some of them had contracted some serious diseases also.

How could that be ? They had avoided those insidious bad habits the other group had succumbed to. What had caused them to become the victims of some of the world's most dangerous diseases ?

The answer is unbelievably simple. They failed on two basic fronts. 1. They neglected to educate themselves on the detriments of some of the most common food additives. 2. They neglected to read the labels of the foods they purchased, refusing to purchase any of the items listing harmful additives. This resulted in their consumption of those harmful additives for extended periods of time. This caused an excessive accumulation of those toxic materials which in turn caused a breakdown in immune function. When immune function decreases, free radical activity increases and your body is left open to attack and disease. When that happens the bad guys win.

Don't you just hate it when you hear about bad guys winning ? You can't help everyone in the world fight the bad guys but you can help yourself, your family, and friends. And the best way to do that is through education. This book will educate you in the various ways to heal and prevent a variety of ailments. And you will accomplish this task using holistic methods. Read the book and keep it handy. You never know when you might need it.

If you recall the previous paragraphs mentioned reading the labels of the food items before you buy. I'm going to give you a classic example of what to look for on those labels and if you detect it, put the item back on the shelf. It's called Sodium Benzoate.

A Dangerous Additive (Sodium Benzoate)

It's supposed to be a safe food additive that's being used to insure our food remains free of fungi and bacteria. It's called Sodium Benzoate but even though it's in our foods and drinks, it doesn't do much to preserve our health. Actually it is seriously detrimental to our health. It can damage our DNA which could lead to degenerative diseases. It can accelerate the aging process and cause liver damage. It can also lead to hyperactivity in children.

Sodium Benzoate on its own is seriously harmful to our health, but mixed with Vitamin C, as in the case with many soft drinks, it turns into Benzene and can become a carcinogen (cancer causing chemical). Add some heat to the mix, like cases of soft drinks sitting in a warehouse in the summertime or in the trunk of your car and the toxic level goes even higher.

The Environmental Protection Agency has classified Benzene as a Class A Carcinogen. Prolonged exposure to a Class A Carcinogen can possibly cause cancer, anemia, bone marrow damage, and a suppressed immune function which can open up a Pandora's Box of potential diseases.

If you don't drink sodas, don't think you've dodged the bullet. Sodium Benzoate is in processed foods, salad dressing, pickles, some fruit juices, and the list goes on and on. The next time you go grocery shopping, take your reading glasses because you'll have to do a lot of label reading to avoid this additive. But take the time to read those labels, your good health depends on it.

Slowing The Aging Process And Living Longer

We would all like to live long healthy lives avoiding the ailments and diseases that seem to plague the elderly. The images of elderly people bent over, limping, on walkers, and in wheelchairs is depressing, especially if that person is a person very dear to you. But what can we do, that's just part of getting old. We have no control over the aging process, right ? Actually that's not entirely true. We do have control over the quality of life we experience as we get older. And a higher quality of life often translates into a longer life span.

Aging, what's that all about anyway ? As we get older our bodies have a tendency to wear out. The human body is like an automobile. It has a large number of moving parts working in unison. And as we all know, an old car does not run as well as a new car.

The same holds true with the human body. The body's moving parts consist of the heart, liver kidneys and many more. As the body gets older, its organs become vulnerable to destructive molecules called free radicals. Free radicals have a tendency to damage and erode our organs making them prone to illness and disease.

One of the best ways to fight free radicals is to eat healthy. Nutritious organic foods are the foundation of a healthy disease free way of life. What we consume in the form of food and liquids goes a long way in determining how healthy we are in our later years.

The old adage "You Are What You Eat" is seriously true. A study revealed that American centenarians (people 100 years or older) eat 2.5 times more vegetables than seniors under the age of 99. And 5 times more vegetables than those in their 40's. It was also revealed that people who ate lots of fresh organic vegetables, didn't smoke or drink excessive amounts of alcohol, have higher antioxidant levels in their bodies and subsequently live longer. What you consume and abstain from consuming plays a major role in determining the quality of your health and ultimately your longevity.

Eating healthy organic foods are fine but there's another equally important aspect of healthy living we should address, and that's supplements. There's compelling evidence that a combination of the amino acid L-Carnitine and the antioxidant Alpha-Lipoic Acid has a revitalizing effect on a person's energy level. They are safe and have no side effects. However, people who have diabetes or have a seizure potential should avoid these two supplements. You don't want to avoid Vitamin C, Resveratrol, or Magnesium however. They rank high on the "to take" list.

Vitamin C enhances the immune system and reduces inflammation. Resveratrol stimulates the SIRT-1 Gene (The Human Anti-Aging Gene). Magnesium helps fortify the length of the protective tips of our chromosomes. All three of these supplements promote longevity and are safe to take. Excessive amounts of Vitamin C can cause diarrhea. What is excessive depends upon the individual, so consider this. If, for example, three caps give you diarrhea, take two and enjoy the added bonus of having regular bowel movements.

You can be disease free, be in tip top physical condition, and it will mean absolutely nothing if your brain is not functioning properly. Your brain is Mission Control for your body. Do not, I repeat, do not underestimate the importance of maintaining a healthy brain. If it is not functioning properly, it can cause a multitude of problems. Every bodily function is controlled by the brain, keep it healthy at all costs. If you don't, you could spend your senior years wasting away in a nursing home.

Let's take a look at some of the steps we can take to prevent the deterioration of our brain cells. This is a subject with which I am intimately familiar. My mother suffered irreversible brain damage resulting from a stroke. I took care of her at home and watched her quality of life slowly slip away. It was heart-breaking to watch knowing there was nothing I could do to stop her regression. I vowed, in my mother's memory, to help as many women as I could to avoid a similar situation.

Senior moments, we've all heard that phrase, what does it mean ? As we get into our later years, our brains, like some of our other organs, don't function as efficiently as they did when we were younger. We misplace items, forget the names of people we know, and sometimes walk into a room and ask ourselves "what did I come in here for ?"

Those situations are what we call Senior Moments. We can minimize or even eliminate senior moments by taking a supplement called Phosphatidyl-Serine (PS). It's a molecule containing the amino acid Serine and essential fatty acids located in virtually every cell membrane. During our younger years our cells had an abundance of PS, all we needed. As we get older, however, our PS levels decline. PS is important because it stimulates the area of the brain responsible for memory, concentration, vocabulary skills, and the ability to learn. PS also has the ability to alleviate the symptoms of Dementia, Depression, Alzheimer's Disease, and the damaging results of Stress. As of this writing, there is no cure for Alzheimer's Disease but PS helps ease some of the symptoms of the disease.

Exercise has long been associated with brain connective function in senior citizens. But please don't wait until you are a senior citizen to start an exercise program. Do it now because exercise increases blood circulation to the brain and all areas of the body. If you have limited mobility, go for a walk. If you haven't exercised in a while, start slowly than increase the tempo gradually. If you are walking, try to walk briskly for 30 minutes 5 days a week.

As you age you are consistently loosing muscle mass. That is often an indirect cause of the many falls seniors experience. A senior can maintain, even increase, muscle mass through diet, supplementation, and weight training. If you decide to include weight training into your regiment, adding protein would definitely be a good idea. Protein not only enhances muscle mass but also contains much of the tissue of your internal organs. A good choice of your protein supplement should be Whey Protein.

Tension Headache

Tension headaches are caused by muscle contractions in the temples or the back of the head. They are usually brought on by stress and could last four hours or even days. This type of headache feels like your head is being compressed from both sides making it almost impossible to sleep. Relief can be achieved by using a cold compress, by massage, or by using acupuncture.

Sinus headaches are the result of congestion or inflammation of the nasal cavity. Symptoms of this problem are a dull ache over the eyes causing irritability and the inability to sleep.

Stress and tension headaches are caused by, as you have probably guessed, stress and tension. But that is where the simplicity ends because each of us, as individuals, have different situations and conditions that cause us to become stressful and tense.

The following are some examples of the causes of stress and tension: Computer eyestrain, pinched nerves, too much caffeine, too much sugar or salt, hypoglycemia (low blood sugar), PMS, artificial sweeteners, a need for a liver detox, candida, a need for a heavy metal detox, a need for a full body detox. You can find more details on detoxification in later chapters of this book. Those and numerous other situations could possibly cause a tension headache.

If you use over the counter drugstore headache drugs on a regular basis, you could be setting yourself up for rebound headaches. Acetaminophen, if combined with alcohol, can cause liver damage. So if you were to have a hangover, don't take Tylenol to get rid of the headache.

If you feel a headache coming on, immediately apply cold, slightly damp black tea bags to your eyes (closed) for 15 minutes or have a cup of black decaf coffee. Consuming Ginger, fresh or supplemental, can often stop a developing headache. Also an ice pack on the back of the neck at the base of the skull is often very effective. But most importantly, if you are not sure why you are getting your headaches, get tested for food allergies. There could be a very simple answer to the problem. It's always easier to prevent a problem than to treat it.

Migraine Headache

When you have a migraine headache, you don't just have a bad headache; you have pain that goes past the traditional 1 to 10 scale. Over 40 million people have migraine headaches and a vast majority are women who have an estrogen dominance.

A typical migraine is the result of the constrictive deformation of the brain, the face, and the scalp resulting in intense throbbing pain that can last for hours or even days. Shortly before an attack the patient will experience an acute sensitivity to odors and light followed by chills, fever, nausea, and vomiting which can last up to 4 days. Those are the symptoms of a "Classic Migraine".

The "Common Migraines" have no sensitivity to light or smell but have the same intense pain. "Cluster Headaches" mean there are two or more spasmodic, extremely painful headaches a day. They cluster in the areas of the forehead and eyes causing visual distortion.

So what can you do to stop the pain ? As you know, it is easier to avoid a problem than to attempt to fix the problem. Food allergies are the major causes of migraines. The most common allergies are to wheat, dairy, caffeine, pickled fish, shellfish, smoked meats, aged cheese, red wine, chocolate, pizza, refined sugar, and Aspartame. One should also avoid grain fed red meats, sodas, soy sauce, citrus, tomatoes, and hard liquor. If you feel an attack coming on start eating high

Magnesium foods like leafy greens or take supplements like Magnesium, Vitamin C, or Bromelain. Keeping these supplements on hand would not be a bad idea. For almost immediate results, give yourself a coffee enema to stimulate the liver and normalize bile activity. The resulting bowel movement could possibly relieve the nausea. You might also consider Gastrodin + Magnesium. Good results have resulted from the absorption of these two supplements.

Solutions For Candida Yeast Infections

Do you suffer from digestive problems like diarrhea and constipation ? Or experience abdominal pains, joint pains, or acid reflux ? Do you have problems with low libido, genital itching, sore throat, or night sweats ? Do you get a burning tongue, sores on the insides of your mouth or tongue way too often ? These conditions frequently become worse when foods high in sugar are consumed or the infected person is located in a damp and moldy area. In extreme cases Candida can travel through the bloodstream infecting the entire body.

Since the symptoms are so numerous, this ailment is frequently misdiagnosed . So the problem frequently goes unchecked for long periods of time. In the mean time your pain and numerous other symptoms get progressively worse. In this chapter you will discover that Candida is known to be the cause of many symptoms including arthritis and even depression. And sugar can make things even worse.

What Is Candida Albicans ?

The Candida yeast feeds on sugar. If the body's pH balance is compromised, the friendly bacteria that normally metabolize sugar cannot function properly and there is a risk of the Candida fungus thriving in the sugar rich environment. Once again we are reminded of the negative role sugar plays with regards to our health.

If you are unfortunate enough to have your mouth infected with the Candida fungus (called Thrush) you will experience painful white sores on your gums and the inside of your cheeks. If a breast feeding infant were to be infected with Oral Thrush it can spread to the mother's nipples and lead to a situation where the mother and the baby continually reinfect each other. Thrush can also infect the baby's buttocks, giving the impression of a diaper rash, possibly resulting in another misdiagnosis.

Women who are pregnant or who use oral contraceptives are often at an increased risk of a yeast infection because there is an increased amount of sugar (Glycogen) in the vagina as a result of a change in hormonal levels. Frequent use of antibiotics, which kill friendly bacteria along with the harmful bacteria are also a common cause of yeast infections.

What causes great concern is that Candida can change from a yeast to a fungus. In it's fungal state Candida becomes invasive with tentacles that penetrate the intestinal tract which could result in Leaky Gut Syndrome and a multitude of food sensitivities. If this were to go unchecked it could potentially infect the whole body.

This is a serious ailment but by no means hopeless. If you are the kind of person I think you are, you are a fighter. So in order to defeat this enemy you must attack with vigor.

Tip #1 Fortify Your Immune System

The enemy (Candida) which thrives in a sugar rich environment preys on those with compromised immune systems. It frequently targets those who use antibiotics, who drink excessive amounts of alcohol, and is often sleep deprived. The enemy frequently targets those who have poor eating habits, who eat fast foods, who eat processed foods and starchy foods which turns to sugar after consumption. You must read those food labels carefully.

Tip #2 How To Prevent An Infection

You can prevent a Candida yeast infection by consuming sugar in moderation. Cutting back on the white stuff alone will not solve the problem, however. You will have to read the labels on everything you purchase at the supermarket because sugar is in almost everything. If you are unfortunate enough to contract this condition, go to your favorite health store and purchase some grapefruit seed extract (not grape seed extract). Add fifteen drops to your favorite juice and consume it three times a day until the symptoms subside.

Tip #3 Test Yourself For A Possible Infection

You can perform a simple test at home to see if you have this problem. Fill a class of water to the brim, work up a big wad of saliva and gently deposit it onto the surface of the water and let it stand for 30 minutes. If, after the 30 minutes has elapsed, the wad of saliva is still intact, you are probably not infected. If, however, the wad breaks up and there are streaks extending downward, you could possibly be infected. To make this test as accurate as possible, it should be performed in the morning immediately after rising. Do not brush your teeth, use mouthwash, or consume anything before performing this test.

Conclusion

To successfully defeat the yeast infection you must go through the following steps.

Step #1

You must kill the yeast. You can do this by diet change which includes a reduction in sugar consumption, a reduced consumption of alcohol (nothing more than one drink for women per day), and the elimination of fast foods and processed foods.

Step #2

You must remove the dead yeast and waste materials from the body using detoxification methods. Detoxification is addressed in the following four chapters of this book. You must also strengthen your digestive system and promote the formation of friendly bacteria in your intestinal tract. You can accomplish this task by taking Probiotic supplements.

Step #3

You must also fortify your immune system by consuming Olive Leaf Extract, Vitamin C, Vitamin E, Vitamin B Complex, and Source Naturals Wellness Formula.

Detoxification

Cleaning The Body's Interior

Purification of the body has been a ritual for thousands of years. It has been the foundation of every sophisticated society and continues to this day. Earlier societies, however, did not have to deal with the pollutants we have to deal with today. It is estimated that we would have to go back 100 years to find foods that are free of the toxins found in today's foods.

We would have to go back even farther to find clean air to breathe and water to drink. So unless you are well over 100 years old, your body has been exposed to a continuous bombardment of pollutants and toxins. The body can repel and extract some of those pollutants but not all of them. So what happens to the toxins the body was unable to extract ?

Our bodies try to protect us from toxic material by setting them aside. It surrounds those toxic materials with mucus and fat in an effort to prevent an imbalance or cause an immune system malfunction. Our bodies store toxic material in fatty tissues, which is a good reason to keep body fat to a minimum. But regardless of your body size, you probably have accumulated significant amounts of toxins in your body. If you take prescription drugs, you have an above average accumulation of drug residue in your body. If you live in a city or near a chemical or industrial plant, you probably have an above average accumulation also.

As time goes on and those accumulations increase, the organs storing those toxins begin to break down. That opens the door for disease to find their way into the body. Detox before that happens. It's easier to prevent a disease than to treat it.

Detoxification Part 2

Every time you take something into your body there is a potentially harmful ingredient coming in. If you are sitting in a traffic jam, the exhaust from the car in front of you is slowly polluting your lungs. Every time you eat processed foods, you are ingesting harmful chemicals used to increase the shelf life of the product. Pollutants are all around us, we can't avoid them. Over time those pollutants start to accumulate in our bodies causing minor and sometimes serious bodily malfunctions. Those malfunctions are your body talking to you. Listen to what your body is saying.

Here are some signs your body has reached a level of toxic intolerance:

1. Frequent headaches, back pain, or joint pain for no logical reason.
2. Sinus or respiratory problems.
3. Coated tongue, body odor, or bad breath.
4. Brittle nails or adult acne.
5. Poor digestion with gas and bloating.
6. Body growths like moles and carbuncles.

You know your body better than anyone else and because these changes come on slowly, they may not get your attention right away. But as the symptoms persist or intensify, they will eventually get your attention. Listen to what your body is trying to tell you. You are the one who is most qualified to translate your body's language. What your body is trying to say is "I'm not feeling to well, please find a way to get these toxins out of me". Your answer should be "OK I'm going to do a detoxification". Also keep in mind, you don't have to be sick or experience negative symptoms to perform a detox on yourself. Detoxification also prevents illness and negative feelings of imbalance. If you have never performed a detox or it has been a long time since your last one, it's time to detox. Love your body, it's your best and oldest friend.

Kidney Detoxification

Your kidneys provide a very important function in your day to day lives. They remove waste elements from your body which keeps your body chemicals in balance and this in turn helps maintain your body's water balance. Exposure to a variety of toxins and drugs can cause serious kidney damage. When your body experiences an invasion of toxins your immune system swings into action by attacking the toxic material, surrounding it with fat and storing it away in one of your body's organs. One of those organs just might be one of the kidneys. As time goes on and those toxic materials start to build up, your kidney function starts to break down and that is when you experience a malfunction of the organ.

Your hands and ankles start to swell and you become short of breath. When the kidneys become overloaded, the toxins then get into the bloodstream which causes even more problems like abdominal pain, chills, fever, back pain, bloating, and nausea. Back pain may come about suddenly and may be intense, located just above the waist and running down the groin.

There are numerous causes of kidney poisoning but if your kidney problems are caused by mercury, prescription or over the counter drugs, then you might try taking Spirulinia or Kidney Detox Plus. Both can be found at health food stores or on their online websites.

Bodywork After A Cleanse

1. Take a daily brisk 30 minute walk to keep the kidneys functioning efficiently.
2. Take a Spirulina or Fleet Enema the day after your cleanse.
3. Take a hot sitz bath for 20 minutes to sweat out toxins.
4. During your sitz bath add 8 to 10 drops of Essential Oils (a combination of 2 or 3 oils like Juniper, Cedarwood, Sandlwood, Lemon, Chamomile, or Eucalyptus) to your bath, stir to evenly distribute the oils.
5. Have someone give you a full body massage to stimulate the circulation.
6. Eat fresh seafood and drink organic Cranberry Juice frequently.
7. Avoid heavy starches, grain fed red meat, prepared meats, dairy foods, salty foods, and fast foods. These all restrict the filtering function of your kidneys.
8. If you are taking medication for your kidney problems, do not stop taking your medication.

Sexually Transmitted Disease (STD)

Herpes Simplex 2 is the most widespread of all the STD's. It affects over 120 million in the USA alone and the number worldwide is increasing faster than we can count. Let's just say the number of new cases each year are in the millions. This is a lifelong infection; once you get it you have it for the rest of your life. There is no cure. If you become infected you will have periods of active and inactive stages. The disease can be passed on to others even during the inactive stages.

Can Babies Become Infected ?

Babies can be infected at birth and since their immune systems are not yet fully developed they can develop brain damage, blindness, even death. And what makes this situation so serious is the fact that over 70% of new infections are transmitted by people who are not aware they have the virus. The herpes virus can be transmitted by kissing, oral sex, intercourse, or the exchange of body fluids. Once you have been infected, outbreaks can be caused by poor diet, emotional distress, overuse of drugs or alcohol, sunburn, the common cold, or a simple fever. Acyclovir, a drug commonly used for treating herpes, can cause numerous side effects that are almost as bad as the disease.

The Initial Outbreak

The first outbreak is usually the most intense. Your glands become swollen and you develop a fever. As your immune system kicks in to fight the infection (assuming your immune system is not depressed) an accumulation of very painful blisters appear on the groin, buttocks, and thighs. If this were not bad enough, flu-like symptoms now appear accompanied by swelling of the groin and the lymph glands. The genitals itch and the blisters start to swell and fester. Intense pain begins to shoot through the thighs and legs. The blisters break in about three days and then slowly heal in about five days. At this point you ask yourself if that seemingly awesome sexual encounter was really worth what you just went through.

If you become infected with the herpes virus you are going to need a lot of help as you try to get through this trying situation. The fact that you are going to have to deal with this problem for the rest of your life may put you into a depressed mental state for a while. But after the initial stage has passed and you realize the worst part is over, that's when you realize it is time to take a positive outlook on the situation and start planning to fight back.

What Is The Treatment ?

I'm sure you are painfully aware that there is no cure, but there are some effective methods of treating the situation. Tea Tree Oil is an herbal antiseptic. During an outbreak you should lightly dab some of it onto the sores and blisters several times a day. If a full strength application causes discomfort, try diluting it with olive oil. Make sure you keep any full strength or diluted strength of Tea Tree Oil away from your eyes. Other herbs good for treating herpes are Echinacea, Red Clover, and St. Johns Wart.

Try to eat the following during outbreaks: Fresh organic vegetables, brown rice, miso soup, and lysine-rich fresh fish. Try to avoid citrus fruits and juices while the virus is active. Apply ice packs to the genital area to reduce swelling and pain. To relieve itching take a warm baking soda or Epsom salt bath. After the bath pat the affected area dry. Never touch the sores with your bare hands, if you do wash your hands immediately and thoroughly.

If you are pregnant and are aware you have genital herpes, make sure your doctor is aware of your situation. If you have an attack near delivery time you may have to have your baby delivered by cesarean section to protect your baby from any contact with the genital lesions.

Your life has changed but it's not the end of the world, and you are a little wiser.

Fibromyalgia

Fibromyalgia is a muscular ailment that affects millions of people, mainly women. Back in the old days it was called Rheumatism. People suffering from this ailment feel pain all over the body and extreme sensitivity is felt when pressure is applied. This ailment is stress related and the cause seems to be a decreased level of Serotonin in the brain. Fibromyalgia symptoms are numerous and diverse, sometimes exhibiting the same symptoms of chronic fatigue syndrome, TMJ, and even rheumatoid arthritis. These are all painful ailments so the next question is what causes Fibromyalgia ? Sadly, the answer is no one is quite sure.

It is believed that Fibromyalgia is caused by a Magnesium deficiency, a virus, immune system failure, or Hypoglycemia. Aside from the pain, some of the other symptoms are dizziness, fatigue, migraine headaches, confusion, diarrhea, and Irritable Bowel Syndrome. Being an overweight smoker increases one's chances of suffering from this ailment. There is no cure but there are treatments. There are drug treatments with a lot of side effects and there are holistic treatments with little or no side effects.

A Holistic Breakthrough

Researchers from Japan have made some noteworthy discoveries in the field of a holistic treatment for Fibromyalgia. Japanese scientists have a history of conducting research on marine plant life. As an island nation, the Japanese turn to the sea and inland waterways for their livelihood which includes, but are not limited to, fishing and marine research. The culmination of their marine research has resulted in the discovery of Chlorella.

It's formal name is Chlorella Pyrenoidosa and it's a form of green fresh water algae that possesses the richest source of plant chlorophyll ever found. It also contains a variety of amino acids, minerals, and vitamins. In detailed sophisticated animal studies, Chlorella has shown a propensity to stimulate immune function, which we all know is the key to maintaining a healthy body. With this fact in mind the researchers set out to test their new product on some of the world's most challenging illnesses like Fibromyalgia.

Extensive clinical trials were conducted and the results, though not overwhelming, were still impressive. It seems as if 72% of the women who participated in the study reported significant improvement in their Fibromyalgia symptoms. And unlike pharmaceuticals, there were no reported side effects.

You can find Chlorella supplements at your local health store or at SunChlorella.com.

The following are some additional holistic treatments:

1. Perform a three day full body detox. The problem could be a build-up of toxins over the years and your body is talking to you the only way it knows how.

2. Avoid caffeine, sugary foods, fatty foods, and grain fed red meat.
3. Take 3-400mg Garlic caps a day (Kyolic Detox Formula) this will maintain aortic flexibility.
4. Take 1-Vitamin B complex 100mg cap a day.
5. Have one 4oz glass of red wine with dinner (Pinot Noir)
6. If you are not exercising, start. Start slowly with a 2 mph walk for 15 minutes and build up to a 3mph walk for 30 minutes. Do this for 5 days a week.
7. Acupuncture has shown good results. It is not painful.
8. Relax, using any method you feel comfortable with.
9. Try visualization. This is done by lying on your back in a comfortable position with your eyes closed and concentrating very hard on picturing yourself free from pain, free from the ailment, enjoying a pain free life with friends and family. We all know the brain controls the body. The visualization method, if done with intense concentration, can possibly work. You don't have to be Rhodes Scholar to make this process work. You do, however, need to be able to mentally block out all outside distractions for about 20 minutes. Results will not happen overnight so stick to it.

YOU CAN DO THIS

Endomedriosis

Endometriosis is a common condition which affects about 16% of the entire female population. And about 50% of the women who have this ailment are infertile. It is estimated that about 2 million women in the UK have Endometriosis and about 5 million women in the United States are afflicted with this ailment.

What Are The Symptoms ?

Are you having intense pain in the uterus and pelvic area before or during menses ? Has that pain continued throughout the menstrual cycle and has there also been during intercourse, excessive bleeding and the passing of shreds and tissue and clots during menses ? If you have difficulty sleeping and experienced painful urination, you may be afflicted with Endometriosis.

Women with this ailment have had to change schedules and miss multiple days of work due to the intense pain, and employers and mainstream medicine have shown little concern or sympathy for the victims of this ailment. Does that make you mad ? It makes me mad. So lets look at some holistic ways to fight this problem.

How To Fight This Problem

If you are seriously concerned about fighting and eliminating this problem, forget about drugs. Their side effects often cause more problems than Endometriosis does.

So if you can't use drugs, what else is there ? You might want to think about trying supplements. Supplements in the form of vitamins, herbs, and minerals are Mother Nature's methods of assisting your body in it's efforts to heal itself with no side effects. So lets get started.

Treatment For Endometriosis

Minerals: Minerals are the building blocks of life, they keep your body pH balanced. To start off, get a bottle of trace minerals, which will give you trace amounts of 70 minerals. Your body requires lesser amounts of trace minerals but they are still essential. A few ounces of liquid trace minerals a day will be sufficient.

Vitamin B Complex: This single capsule includes vitamin B6 which has proven to significantly reduce the intensity of menstrual pains. The B Vitamins are extremely important because the liver requires them to convert excess estrogen in weaker and less menacing forms.

Vitamin E: This vitamin has a good track record when it comes to relieving menstrual cramps in women with Endometriosis. Start out with a dosage of 400IU and increase to 800IU if necessary.

Vitamin C with Bioflavonoids: This vitamin is one of the major antioxidants and plays a major role in supporting an efficient immune system. In doing so it allows your body to recognize and kill Endometrial patches as they occur. The addition of Bioflavonoids are helpful with regards to pain management during the time of the menstrual cycle allowing the smooth muscles to relax and prevent inflammation.

Magnesium: This mineral needs to be consumed in larger than trace quantities. It acts as a muscle relaxer resulting in a positive effect on painful periods and back pain. Take 250mg-500mg a day. Also for every 250mg of Magnesium take 500mg of Calcium.

This is not going to be an overnight fix. It should take approximately three months to achieve maximum effectiveness. Don't give up.

Conclusion

Having a highly functional immune system is the best way to defeat Endometriosis. You can accomplish this by choosing not to smoke and consuming alcohol in moderation (one drink a day). You can also fortify your immune system by implementing a low fat dairy free diet. This will decrease estrogen production. Enhance that low fat diet by consuming fresh organic fruits and vegetables. And finally, avoid UDT's. They are major contributors to an Endometriosis infection.

Stroke

Why It Happens And How To Prevent It

Some of the people who were lucky enough to experience the symptoms of a stroke and live to tell about it say they had no prior warning, It seemed that in an instant, something went seriously wrong.

Even though the attack seemed to happen in an instant, the cause of that devastating event had been building up for years. When blood, and the oxygen and nutrients in the blood, are blocked from reaching the brain, a stroke occurs. The blockage is usually caused by a blood clot blocking an artery in or leading to the brain. A stroke can also happen if an artery bursts, resulting in a loss of blood.

If you have high blood pressure, high cholesterol, or diabetes, you have an increased risk of having a stroke. You can reduce your risk significantly by simply choosing healthy foods. You are what you eat.

How To Lower Your Blood Pressure

If you are serious about lowering your blood pressure and you are overweight, start by losing those extra pounds. Being overweight raises your risk of having a stroke by 75%. Being obese raises your risk of having a stroke by 100%. Researchers found that overweight women were more likely to have high blood pressure, diabetes, and high cholesterol than their normal weight counterparts.

Researchers also found that eating two to three servings of fruits and vegetables a day reduced your potential for having a stroke by 23%. Fruits and vegetables are high in fiber content which is instrumental in the lowering of cholesterol. Because of this reduction in cholesterol, (total and LDL), artery walls have less plaque, which restricts and sometimes totally blocks, blood flow to the brain. Eat those organic fruits and vegetables, especially garlic, carrots, onions, broccoli, oranges, red grapes, and leafy greens.

Preventing High Blood Pressure

High blood pressure (hypertension) has become a major health concern in today's stressful fast paced society. One third of Americans have high blood pressure and as more women have entered the fast paced corporate environment, more women are starting to experience high blood pressure.

Actually, about half of those with high blood pressure are not even aware they have the condition. That's serious because high blood pressure causes more than 70,000 deaths a year and is directly related to 350,000 additional deaths from stroke. It is commonly called the "silent killer" because in many cases there are no symptoms. But it is a serious condition that can increase the potential for heart attack, heart failure, and kidney malfunction. It can also cause hardening of the arteries, damage to the heart, and damage to the blood vessels.

How Do We Get High Blood Pressure ?

Over time, our consumption of high fat meals has resulted in clogging of our arteries plus an accumulation of fat. This condition is caused by a deficiency of calcium, magnesium, and fiber. Also our propensity for consuming fast foods and our lack of exercise are not helping the situation. But fast foods are not the only villains. There are other villains like a high sugar diet, grain fed red meat, excessive salt, excessive alcohol, smoking, being around smokers, and too much caffeine. All these contribute to thickened blood with excessive mucous and waste, plus insulin resistance resulting from poor sugar metabolism. It has been proven through extensive research that people with high blood pressure who make a concerted effort to make healthy lifestyle changes have shown more improvement than their counterparts who relied on blood pressure prescription drugs. Those who follow a vegetarian diet have fewer high blood pressure issues also.

If the idea of following a vegetarian diet does not appeal to you and you want to avoid prescription drugs (A Good Idea), try supplements. Try Potassium 300mg, Garlic (Kyolic Formula 105 2 caps), Hawthorn 510mg x 2, Reishi Mushroom 600mg x 2, Olive Leaf Extract 500mg x 2, and Rosemary 400mg x 2. Start with one and increase by one until you find the right combination.

What Does 120 Over 80 Mean ?

The ideal blood pressure is 120 over 80. The 120 is called the systolic and represents the pressure exerted when the heart pumps. The 80 is called the diastolic and that represents the residual pressure exerted when the heart rests between beats. A reading of 140 over 90 is classified as hypertension. If the diastolic (bottom number) goes over 105, severe hypertension is indicated. When you go to the doctor's office, the standard procedure is for the nurse to check your blood pressure.

So how often do you go to the doctor's office ? Women should keep regular tabs on their blood pressure. Don't wait for the doctor's nurse to check it, check it yourself.

Testing Your Blood Pressure At Home

Home blood pressure kits can be purchased at your local drug store or even at your local supermarket. Home blood pressure kits range in price from $20.00 to about $75.00, they are more accurate as the price goes up. If you elect to purchase the least expensive kit, take it to the doctor's office the next time you go and compare his reading with you home kit. Actually testing your blood pressure at home is more reliable than testing at the doctor's office because people often become anxious when visiting a doctor's office which would result in a higher than normal reading. Also driving to the doctor's office in congested traffic will cause your blood pressure to rise. When you test yourself at home you are more relaxed and a more accurate reading can be achieved.

Conclusion

A high percentage of high blood pressure cases are preventable without the use of drugs. A good fat free and low salt diet can be highly effective in controlling high blood pressure. Also drinking 8-8oz glasses of steam distilled bottled water a day will balance your body salt. When your body feels dehydrated, it reacts by retaining sodium to reduce any further water loss which starts an endless cycle of craving for salt which causes the blood pressure to rise.

Heart Attack

Heart attacks used to be a male problem but that's not the case anymore. Women are now having heart attacks at an increasing rate resulting in almost 50% of all heart attacks. That's right, the percentage of male and female heart attacks is now dead even. And to make matters even worse, 44% of women die within a year of their attacks. Only 27% of men die with a year of their attacks. If that doesn't get your attention, consider this. On a yearly basis, twice as many women die from heart attacks as die from all forms of cancer combined.

What Are The Signs Of A Possible Attack ?

Men and women have different warning signs of an impending heart attack. It's wise not to ignore any chest pain or discomfort but the common warning signs we have all heard about are basically signs men should observe. A recent study revealed some disturbing facts. It seems as if only 29% of female heart attack victims experienced the intense chest pains that are common in male heart attacks. Because of this, many women are unaware of the gravity of their condition and subsequently delay treatment. This decision all too often proves fatal.

What Signs Should A Woman Look For ?

By all means observe the symptoms men look for. But

also become aware of the symptoms specific to a woman's situation. Your life may depend on it. The following are symptoms that can appear up to one month before an attack.

- Unusual fatigue that can't be explained.
- Anxiety accompanied by poor sleep patterns.
- Excessive weakness and dizziness (Attack Imminent).
- Shortness of breath with or without pain.
- Shortness of breath plus palpitations and cold sweats (Attack Imminent).

If You Experience One Or More Signs, What Should You Do ?

If you experience any of the signs mentioned above seek emergency help at once. While you are waiting for emergency help to arrive, observe the following:

If you are unable to verbally correspond with the 911 operator, make some sounds of distress like moans or groans. This will indicate to the 911 operator that this is not a prank call. Do not hang up after. That will allow the call to be traced.

If you were able to verbally correspond with the 911 operator, hang up after you have completed the conversation. Then immediately call a friend or relative who can get to your location quickly to render assistance if needed.

If you have nitroglycerin tablets, take one every five minutes, three maximum. If you have aspirin, take one and chew it. This can possibly prevent a blood clot.

Perform a coughing maneuver called Cough CPR which consists of continuous vigorous coughing. This could possibly prevent you from losing consciousness.

If a companion is with you, have them check your pulse and respiration at frequent intervals. If your breathing or pulse stops your companion should immediately perform CPR until breathing is restored or the ambulance arrives.

How To Become Heart Healthy And Avoid A heart Attack

One of the best ways to become heart healthy is to by improving your diet. The following are a few methods to assist you in your efforts to make your heart healthier and stronger.

If you have a juicer, drink some fresh fruit and vegetable juice from organic produce. If you don't have a juicer try some commercial organic bottled juices. Also try to consume about 64 oz of steam distilled water per day.

Avoid sugar, salt, and anything produced from white flour. Refined sugars promote negative reactions in all of your body's cells.

Avoid excessive consumption of alcohol, it has a negative effect on your heart. For a woman, excessive use is classified as anything over one drink a day.

The supplements Coenzyme Q10, Carnitine, Flax, Magnesium, Vitamin C, Vitamin E, and Vitamin B complex are instrumental in the prevention of cardiac arrhythmia and heart attack. Carnitine protects the heart from damage due to poor circulation or partial blockage of the arteries. Taking the supplements DHA and EPA also help to reduce the risk of having a heart attack. They also reduce your chances of dying from a variety of ailments, including heart disease.

Conclusion

The heart muscle pumps blood to all areas of the body. It is comprised of four separate chambers, the right and left atria and the right and left ventricles. Between these four chambers are valves that allow blood to flow in a forward direction only. With each beat of the heart the right ventricle forces deoxygenated blood into the lungs and the left ventricle pumps oxygenated blood into the arteries for circulation throughout the body.

Your heart depends on oxygenated blood coming to it from the arteries around the heart (coronary arteries) for essential oxygen and nutrients. If the coronary arteries become constricted the heart will be deprived of much need oxygen resulting in a heart attack causing the death of cardiac tissue. When the blood supply to the heart is reduced or stopped, the heart is deprived of essential oxygen and if blood flow is not restored quickly (within minutes) portions of the heart deteriorate and die resulting in permanent damage to your heart.

Heart attacks have become a serious problem for women. A woman is 50% more likely to die from a heart attack than a man. Why? Because women are having heart attacks at older ages when their immune systems are less efficient due to the aging process. The chain reaction continues when her arteries are less able to adjust to the partial death of the heart muscle caused by the heart attack. Death is often the end result.

Heart attacks are directly related to a variety of other conditions like arteriosclerosis, circulatory problems, high blood pressure, high cholesterol, and cardiovascular disorders like Angina and Arrhythmia.

People with high blood pressure should avoid cold weather climates. The cold weather could possibly cause an increase in blood pressure putting the woman at a greater risk for a heart attack.

Many ailments have the symptoms that resemble a woman's heart attack symptoms such as a gallbladder attack or Fibromyalgia which causes chest pain. Even unexplained symptoms should be thoroughly checked. Remember some signs of an impending heart attack for a woman appear well in advance of the actual attack.

Stress

How is your life going these days ? Been under any stress lately ? It doesn't matter whether your answer is yes or no the, the real answer is yes. We are all aware of the negative situations that become stressful like financial problems, divorce, chronic pain, rush hour traffic, problem teenagers and many other similar situations. But there are actually positive situations that can cause stress like preparing for a dinner party, starting a new job, the birth of your first child, getting married, and other similar happy events. All of these situations in both negative and positive categories have a tendency to generate a degree of worry, and worry produces stress.

Stress can cause headaches, memory loss, low self-esteem, high blood pressure, digestive problems, insomnia, cancer, anxiety and depression. Stress also causes your immune system to become less effective or even ineffective. If that were to happen, you would become vulnerable to a myriad of ailments and diseases.

Stress is frequently looked upon as a psychological problem but it can cause some serious problems. Your body often responds to stress with a variety of physiological changes such as the secretion of adrenaline, greater muscle tension, accelerated heart beat, and the elevation of blood pressure. Digestion is adversely effected, cholesterol levels increase, and blood consistency changes making it more prone to clotting. This results in an increased risk of a heart attack and stroke.

Almost all of your bodily functions and the associated organs react to stress. The pituitary gland increases the production of hormones that inhibit the function of your immune system. The resulting physical change is called the fight or flight response where the body's organs prepare for physical battle or physical retreat. Most of the time neither occasion arises but your body remains in a state of stressful readiness.

When your body is under stress it cannot absorb nutrients well due to the complex physical reactions that take place. When your body is under prolonged stress it becomes seriously deficient in numerous nutrients and unable to replace them in a timely manner. One of the more important nutrients that become depleted is Vitamin B Complex. The B Complex vitamins are instrumental in the proper functioning of the nervous system and electrolytes, which become depleted as a result of your body's response to stress. Stress also promotes the formation of free radicals that can damage body tissues and membranes.

Obsessive compulsive disorder, phobic disorders, panic attacks, post traumatic stress disorders, and anxiety are some of the more serious emotional problems related to stress.

A common theory is that stress related symptoms are attributed to a malfunction of the nervous system. And that's true, to a certain extent. Actually stress usually does affect the parts of the body that are linked to the nervous system like the digestive organs. Stressful symptoms related to the digestive organs could appear as irritable bowel syndrome or even an ulcer. If that type of stress is not addressed promptly, more serious illnesses could possibly result.

Stress can be classified as acute or long term. Of those two classifications, long term is the most dangerous. When stress continues over a long term, your body's immune response declines making you susceptible to illness and retards any healing process that may be required later.

Stress is probably one of the most dangerous enemies of longevity and overall health you will encounter. It can cause hormonal damage within your body that can cause brain damage, heart damage, damage to your vascular system, and even elevate your blood pressure. If you have existing problems like herpes, asthma, or allergies, stress will make them worse and hinder the recovery from just about any illness you may encounter in the future.

Actually all stress is not bad. Mother Nature knew there would be times when we would encounter imminent dangerous situations in our lives and we would need to properly address the situation to avoid serious injury or even death.

Here's An Example

Lets say you are on an African Safari, you're on foot and a long way from your vehicle. Off in the distance a ferocious beast pictures you as its next meal and begins to charge you. This is definitely a stressful situation and and the fight or flight scenario kicks in.

Do you fight ? Maybe not, the beast is a good distance away, you may miss the shot. Do you flee? That's not a good idea either. The vehicle is too far and a four legged animal will overtake a two legged human in a very short distance.

You decide to fight. So you aim your high powered rifle and shoot. And you miss. The beast is getting closer, your heart is beating faster, beads of sweat appear on your face. You shoot again and you miss again. You are about to panic. You realize that if you could not survive the flight scenario a minute ago you certainly could not survive now. So you stand your ground and aim your final shot. You realize if you miss this time you will die a very painful death. So you take a deep breath steady your rifle and take your final shot. Your aim is true and the threat to your life has ended.

How Did Mother Nature Prepare You For This Event ?

When your heart beat increased, it increased the flow of blood to your brain allowing you to logically asses the situation. Should I fight or flee ? You began to sweat even though the temperature remained the same. As the sweat began to evaporate it presented a cooling effect on your body allowing you to remain calm for the final and decisive shot. Since Mother Nature had no way of knowing whether you would fight or flee, she prepared you for both situations. However, Mother Nature prepared you for occasional stressful situations, not continuous situations like driving in rush hour traffic five days a week or having to listen to household noise every day.

How Can We Address Stress ?

What you eat has a lot to do with the amount of stress you have to deal with. Try to consume a diet composed of 50% to 70% raw foods like fresh organic fruits and vegetables. Also try to include valuable vitamin and mineral supplements like Vitamin C with Bioflavonoids because they are rich in Flavonoids, the mortal enemy of the free radical. If you chose not to eat your fruits and vegetables raw, try steaming them lightly.

What To Avoid

By all means, avoid processed foods, carbonated soft drinks, especially colas, artificial sweeteners, fried foods, junk foods, and white flour products.

Regular Exercise Is Important

Some people like to walk early in the morning, others like to jog with a partner. Still others like to play tennis or golf on the weekends. Any type of exercise will do as long as you do it on a daily basis, or at least three to five days a week. If you are a once a week tennis player or golfer, do some regular walking or jogging in between.

Learn To Relax

A good way to do this is by visualization. This is a process where you lie on your back in a totally quiet setting with your eyes closed. And you mentally picture yourself free of stress. You visualize yourself in a happy state of mind doing fun and relaxing things. Stay in this state of visualization for approximately thirty minutes. At first you may have difficulty staying mentally focused, but the more you do it the easier it will become. Start out with a ten minute session and gradually increase your times until you get to your thirty minute goal. Do this once or twice a day.

Try some aromatherapy. No one needs to tell you about aromatherapy, you apply it every time you place a dab of perfume or scented oil on your body. You enjoy the aroma and so does anyone who comes close to you. So why not apply some of that "feel good" aroma to yourself ?

There are highly concentrated distilled plant essences called essential oils that specifically target a variety of ailments. The oils targeting stress are Lavender, Sandlewood, and Chamomile. They come in very small bottles of .5oz and each drop of essential oil is highly concentrated.

There are two ways to benefit from aroma therapy. You can simply remove the bottlecap and inhale the aroma from the bottle, or you can place a drop or two on your pillow at bedtime. If either of those methods are not practical for your situation feel free to improvise. If you feel as if your stress has gotten out of control and you can no longer handle it on your own, consider seeking outside help.

Conclusion

The situation that ranked the highest with regards to stress was the death of a loved one. Followed by divorce, marriage, personal illness, financial problems, teenage parenting, and so on. Studies have discovered that the more stress a person is under, the greater their chances of encountering a serious illness. Mental problems often lead to physical problems.

Addressing stress in our younger population should be high on your priority list. Peer pressure, problems at school both socially and academically, bullying both cyber and physical, and sexual issues can lead to anxiety in young children and adolescents. They often act out their feelings of stress in ways adults find hard to understand. Be patient with them.

It has been discovered that stress can cause an increase in allergic reactions. You don't have to be a neurologist to figure that one out. If stress can negatively affect so many bodily functions, the sleep process is probably one of those functions, and you would be right. And if you have ever been deprived of sleep, you are painfully aware of the stress it can cause. Sleep deprivation can cause a significant release of the stress hormones Cortisol and Adrenaline which can negatively affect your brain and your waistline. So the bottom line is there is solid evidence connecting sleep deprivation to stress.

One of the best ways to curtailing your stress is to do some basic things to relax like going for a walk in a relaxing atmosphere, watch a sunset, embrace your pet, take a warm bath surrounded by scented candles providing the only light as you listen to some soft music.

Supplements For Stress Relief

Serotonin is the Neuro Chemical associated with the feelings of relaxation and contentment. Your body produces Serotonin from Tryptophan, an amino acid, which converts to 5-HTP which then becomes Serotonin. Serotonin is reported to calm the mind and make sleep easier and more restful. Start with the lowest dosage and work your way up to a point with which you are comfortable. Do not go over 300mg.

L-Theanine is an amino acid that produces a relaxing effect and it's found in capsule form and it's also found in Green Tea. L-Theanine is also helpful in improving mood and increasing a state of relaxation. If you decide to drink the tea you will need to drink three cups a day. If you choose the supplement, follow the dosage directions on the container.

Breast Cancer

Every year almost a quarter of a million women learn that they have invasive breast cancer. About 58,000 of those will learn that they have contracted early cases of the disease, and about 45,000 will actually die from the disease.

Some women are so fearful of this disease that some are electing to have double mastectomies in an all-out effort to eliminate a potential infection. And even though the statistics are a bit discouraging, there are signs of hope with regards to the prevention of this disease. And, as you might expect, it's not a new drug or surgical procedure. It comes from the head of the family, Mother Nature.

It's estimated that around 50% of the cancer cases could be cured by simply making a few changes in diet and lifestyle. That alone could possibly save the lives of about 22,000 women a year, one of them could be you or someone you love.

The use of specific means in an effort to prevent cancer from developing is called chemoprevention. If properly applied, it could possibly eliminate pre-malignant cells, interfere with the progression of normal cells into marauding tumors, and eventually stop a cancer before it reaches a size that produces detectable symptoms.

Research into this field has produced some significant and positive results. For example, you can reduce your chances of contracting cancer by adding Calcium, Vitamin D3, and Selenium to your supplement routine. And these three supplements are just the tip of the iceberg when it comes to the supplements that will enhance your chemoprevention of breast cancer. In the following paragraphs I will evaluate some extremely encouraging discoveries in the field of breast cancer preventive supplementation.

Epigenetics, A New Science

Breast cancer has received a lot of attention from the medical and holistic communities lately and all of that attention has spawned a new science called Epigenetics. This new science has demonstrated how we have a significant amount of control of whether we get cancer or avoid it. It's the study of long lasting changes in gene function that don't necessarily involve changes in gene structure. We have learned, from Epigenetics, that we can use items like nutrients and supplements to turn genes on and off.

If an activated gene is a gene that prevents cell reproduction or one that stimulates the destruction of defective sells, the Epigenetic changes become capable of blocking the development of a cancerous cell.

So we're finally getting some much needed information on how nutrients and supplements can alter the way breast cancer cells mature and multiply. Knowing this we have also become aware of what prevents cancer cells from multiplying.

The science of Epigenetics has, through extensive research and testing, come up with a list of supplements that can possibly reduce the risk of contracting breast cancer. The next seven paragraphs will list the supplements that can be instrumental in approaching and ultimately defeating various stages of breast cancer development.

Supplements That Prevent DNA Damage

Like most cancers, breast cancer begins with the change in the DNA of a cell. The resulting DNA damage can cause a cell to become malignant. The resulting transformation can cause a tumor impressor gene to become activated allowing unrestricted cell multiplication. That's the bad news. The good news is there are several nutrients that can prevent the DNA damage which leads to the formation of a cancerous cell. The following is a list of those nutrients.

Coenzyme Q10

Curcumin

Green Tea Polyphenols

Lycopene

Melatonin

Resveratrol

Selenium

Soy with Genistein and Diadzein

Supplements That Change Malignant Cells Back To Healthy Cells

There are situations where malignant cells have been reversed, but there is still a chance that the reversal cannot become permanent. The following supplements can help to solidify that reversal.

Vitamin D3

N-Acetylcysteine (NAC)

Conjugated Linoleic Acid (CLA)

Supplements That Prevent Cell Multiplication

One of cancer's best known, and infamous features is it's ability to multiply large numbers of cancerous cells. There are several supplements that have the capability of slowing or even stopping the continuous cycle of cell multiplication and growth. The following is a list of those supplements.

Selenium

Resveratrol

Melatonin

Apigenium

Pterostilbene

Supplements That Cause The Death Of Cancer Cells

Apoptosis is the natural process of controlling cell multiplication. Non cancerous cells have the unique ability to self-destruct if they obtain signals that they are mutiplying too fast. If the cells are malignant, however, they no longer have that characteristic which contributes to their significant growth rate. Several supplements have the ability to restore the breast cancer cell's ability to perish by Apoptosis. They are as follows.

Vitamin D3

Curcumin

Green Tea

Pomegranate

Quercetin

Soy with Genistein and Diadzein

Supplements That Curtail Estrogen Production

An enzyme called Aromatase is responsible for the production of estrogen in the body's tissue, including the cells in your breast. So restricting Aromatase's activity is an important means of curtailing the growth of 71% of estrogen dependent breast cancer cases. The supplements capable of achieving this are as follows.

Vitamin D3

Pomegranate

Melatonin

Hops

Grape Seed Extract

Supplements That Stop The Supply Of Blood
To Growing Tumors

When a cancer cell develops into it's rapid growth phase, it requires a significant amount of blood to sustain that rapid growth. Tumor cells have the unique ability to produce new blood vessels to accommodate the increased blood flow to the area. The cessation of blood flow to the tumor would mean the tumor would ultimately die. The following are the supplements capable of cutting off the flow of blood to a tumor.

Vitamin D3

Coenzyme Q10

Melatonin

Omega 3 Fatty Acids

Green Tea

Quercetin

Pomegranate

Soy with Genistein and Diadzein

Supplements That Prevent Tumors From Spreading

Growing tumors have developed a bad habit of invading local and regional tissues and to fertilize other areas with malignant tissues. This is made possible when the tumors increase the production of protein liquefying enzymes known as Matrix Metallo Proteinases (MMPs). Epigenetic changes that prevent the tumor's production of MMPs are brought about by the following supplements.

Coenzyme Q10
Curcumin
Melatonin
Green Tea Polyphenols
Soy with Genistein and Diadzein

Breast Cancer, The Basics

By the time breast cancer has been detected, a complex series of events have already occurred. Events that have turned a normal healthy cell into an unhealthy cancerous cell. These events have caused cancer to occur when the cell replication process goes hay-wire.

In a healthy body, excessive cell replication is tightly controlled by genetic signals from genes known as tumor suppressors and suicide genes. A tumor suppressor is activated when it responds to an abnormal signal, it prevents cell division from getting out of control. Also, in a similar situation, the activation of a suicide gene ignites a programed form of cellular death called Apoptosis.

So the bottom line is this. Cancer develops when genes within your tissues express themselves adversely. An example of expressing themselves adversely would be when the function of a gene changes, whether it be the activation of cancer producing genes or the deactivation of cancer suppressing genes.

Conclusion

The leading female malignancy is breast cancer and it seems as if all the efforts on this subject from mainstream medicine has been channeled towards treatment after the disease has taken hold .

However there are numerous supplements readily available at health stores, on line, and even at supermarkets that accomplish such tasks as preventing tumors from spreading, cutting off the blood supply of existing tumors, changing malignant cells back to healthy cells, and numerous other fetes. But most importantly, there are supplements that prevent DNA damage. These supplements accomplish these fetes by manipulating your genes in a positive way. So positive they could quite possibly help you erase the "C" word from your vocabulary.

Obesity

Have you tried several diets without success ? Or maybe you have tried a diet with moderate success only to feel the disappointment of gaining those lost pounds back a short time later. Don't feel bad, it happens more often than you think.

If you were overweight as a child you probably had the misfortune of being teased and ridiculed because of your inability to attain that "Barbie" look. After you reached adulthood the teasing may have stopped but the weight issue didn't. When you were a child, your weight issues probably effected your self-esteem. Now that you are older you could still be facing low self-esteem, depression, and some other serious health issues. Diseases like high blood pressure, heart disease, joint pain, osteoarthritis, sleep apnea, and cancer are more prevalent in an overweight person.

The numbers on the scale are only part of the issue, however. More important than your weight is the percentage of body fat. Women naturally have a higher percentage of body fat compared to that of a man. A woman's body is designed to carry a larger portion of fatty tissue to ensure that there is sufficient fuel for a potential pregnancy and nursing in case of a potential food shortage. But as excessive fat accumulates, it starts to squeeze into the space occupied by your internal organs. This compression can eventually cause the compressed organs to function at a decreased capacity, opening the door for possible diseases of the organs.

So, as you can see, being overweight can effect more than your looks and your self-esteem. It can effect your health and your quality of life.

Some of the most common causes of obesity are poor diet (over eating or eating excessive amounts of calories) and insufficient exercise. Diabetes and glandular malfunctions can also be contributors to this ailment. But there are ways to beat the overweight issue, natural ways that don't involve pharmaceuticals and their ever present side effects. The following are some natural approaches to losing weight.

Fucothin Green

Fucothin Green is a combination of two highly effective supplements named Xanthigen and Svetol Green Coffee Bean Extract. On their own, they are effective weight loss supplements. Combined they are even more effective. Lets take a look at these two supplements.

Xanthigen is a product of a brown seaweed which is instrumental in weight management and the effective function of your liver. It contains Fucoxanthin, which is a unique and widely researched compound.

Svetol Green Coffee Bean Extract is one of the newest weight loss supplements on the market. Even though it's made from coffee beans it's almost caffeine free and provides an impressive weight management potential.

Together these two provide an effective weight loss supplement called Fucothin Green.

Safflower Oil

Research at a major university found that among post-menopausal women who have type-2 diabetes, adding Safflower Oil to their diet caused a reduction in belly fat by 6% over a four month span. Combining Safflower Oil with a regular moderate exercise program could produce even better results.

Conjugated Linoleic Acid (CLA)

CLA is a healthy fat found in organic beef which promotes the breakdown and burning of fat. It has a tendency to reduce the volume of stored fat while helping to preserve muscle. Tonalin, a similar form of CLA, has been found to produce fat loss and also prevents the regaining of weight previously lost.

Special Fibers

Glucomannan and PGX are two special fiber supplements that promote weight loss. Minute quantities of these two supplements expand in your stomach causing you to feel full after eating small quantities of food. You should take this supplement with 8 to12 oz of water 5 to 10 minutes before eating every meal.

Conclusion

Obesity is a serious health issue. At one time it was looked upon as the failings of a person with low self-esteem. We now classify it as a disease because it has reached epidemic proportions in the United States, Europe, Australia, Asia, and South America.

The, so called, experts have differing opinions on how and why people become overweight. But they basically agree that the key to losing weight is to eat less and exercise more. Your body has to burn more calories than it takes in.

To lose weight you will have to go through two phases . Phase one will be the active weight loss phase and phase two will be the weight maintenance phase.

In Phase One you should set your goal to lose 10% of your body weight in the next three to four months. You can do this by reducing your calorie intake to a point where you feel comfortable. You will not succeed if you are not comfortable with your choice of diet program.

In Phase Two, the maintenance phase, which should last for eight to nine months, your ultimate goal should be to stabilize your current weight. You can do this by exercising regularly and keeping close tabs on your caloric intake so you don't regain the weight you previously lost in Phase One. Once the eight to nine month phase has ended start the entire two phase cycle again.

One very important item to consider is your choice of diet. Many people base their choice on the predictions of success and the estimated amount of weight that will be lost. Before you commit to a program, try to dig deeper into the inner workings of that particular program. Find out what types of foods you will be limited to eating and which foods you will be restricted from eating. Make your choice wisely because the program you ultimately choose will be an integral part of your life for a long time.

Depression

Have you been experiencing feelings of inadequacy lately ? Have you lost interest in the things that used to bring pleasure to your life? These and numerous others are some of the early symptoms of depression, and women experience symptoms of depression more than men. There are multitudes of symptoms like the inability to experience pleasure, excessive sleeping, quickness to anger, thoughts of suicide, unexplained headaches and backaches, showing little or no emotion, and numerous others.

Depression effects more than 20% of the American population over the age of eighteen every year. In the United States, it's classified as one of the most common medical issues. This is a medical issue that effects your entire body. It effects the way you feel about yourself, the way you feel about other people, even the way you think. There is no time limit with regards to the length of time the symptoms will last. They can last for days, weeks, or even years.

There are several types of depression and the symptoms vary with regards to frequency, severity, and intensity. The categories of depression can be broken down into three divisions, Chronic Depression, Dysthymic Disorder, and Bipolar Depression. There are variations within these major categories with regards to severity, frequency, and the intensity of symptoms.

Chronic Depression

Chronic Depression, is a milder form of depression that exhibits persistent symptoms that can possibly last for extended periods of time, even for years. This milder form of depression rarely interferes with a person's everyday activities but these people rarely feel like they are functioning at their fullest potential. They always feel like there is something missing but can't quite figure out what it is.

Dysthymia Disorder

The most common form of depression is a chronic mild form called Dysthymia. It consists of long term and repetitive depressive symptoms. These symptoms are far from debilitating but prevent a person from leading a normal life. They also interfere with a person's social life and their ability to enjoy themselves. Pleasure is not a part of a depressed person's life. This type of depression frequently results from negative thinking habits.

For those who live in colder climates, the winter months with their cold dark days present a breeding ground for depression. This type of depression is known as seasonal affective disorder (SAD). It's a well documented fact that women are afflicted with this disorder more than men. People with SAD are inclined to gain weight, suffer anxiety attacks, sleep too much, and have low energy levels. The suicide rate generally increases during this time of year.

It is the opinion of the American Psychiatric Society that the majority of depression cases can be treated effectively but 81% of those cases do not get the help they need. Why? There are numerous reasons. Many people are ashamed of their conditions and choose to remain in seclusion. Frequently, people suffering from depression do not seek help until they are near a breaking point. Tragically, an estimated 16% of the more serious cases end in a successful suicide attempt. The ultimate healing approach for a person suffering from depression is strong loyal support from friends and family. With their support and understanding and their ability to influence the patient to seek professional help, serious progress can be made.

Bipolar Disorder

A Bipolar Mood Disorder is slightly different from the classic form of depression. It starts out as a basic form of depression and gradually progresses into alternating states of depression and mania (excessive excitement and enthusiasm). A person with a severe case can go from being in misery and suicidal to feeling dangerously invincible and extremely euphoric.

People with Bipolar Disorder often withdraw from society, become very pessimistic, become extremely irritable, and become enraged at the slightest provocation. People with this disorder are capable of going to extremes from both ends of the spectrum.

Symptoms of Bipolar Disorder can vary extremely. Both depression and elation can vary in intensity and length. A person's symptoms can fluctuate from highs to lows numerous times over periods of days, weeks, and even years. People with this type of depression often sleep for extended periods of time, often rarely getting out of bed. Since they stay in bed for extended periods of time, it's not long before they lose their jobs, and their social lives eventually suffer also.

Then there are others who go to work regularly, have seemingly normal social lives, but inwardly feel a profound sadness resulting in their inability to experience anything pleasurable.

Treatment For Depression

Fifteen years ago, after extensive testing, a new dietary supplement called SAM-e was introduced to the public. It was promoted as a supplement that could quite possibly relieve the symptoms of depression and even arthritis. The print media picked up on all the publicity and added to the frenzy by publicizing numerous articles in some of the most popular magazines which just added to the popularity of this "new" supplement.

All that publicity prompted the US Department of Health and Human Services to evaluate the supplement. After a thorough evaluation they published their findings in an

Evidence Report. The report came to the conclusion that SAM-e was just as effective at treating depression as the most commonly prescribed drugs on the market (minus the numerous side effects).

Vitamin B Complex is essential for the elevation of mood disorders, especially Bipolar Disorder. It seems as if those with Bipolar Disorder have a deficiency of the B Vitamins. Whenever possible, take your your supplements in the sub-lingual form (under the tongue) since it offers the best method of absorption into your system. Try to take 100mg three times a day for Bipolar treatment. Vitamin B Complex not only helps improve the condition of Bipolar Disorder but it also stimulates memory function and promotes longevity. After your depression has ceased, it might be a good idea to continue taking the Vitamin B Complex, 100mg once a day should be sufficient.

Conclusion

There are three major categories of depression, Chronic Depression, Dysthymic Disorder, and Bipolar Disorder and numerous sub-categories of all three. The causes are unknown but it's estimated that heredity, diet, food allergies, a depressed immune system, vitamin and mineral deficiencies play a major role.

The common pharmaceuticals prescribed for depression offer an objectionable array of side effects which has caused those who suffer from depression to seek alternative solutions. One of those alternative solutions comes in the form of vitamin, mineral, and herbal supplementation. Vitamin B12, Vitamin B Complex, SAM-e, and Taurine are a few of the major players in this category. Check them out to find out which are best for your specific needs.

Lupus

If you have been having arthritic like pain with swelling of your fingers, toes, and other joints, it may not be arthritis. If, after further investigation, you notice a red rash across your facial cheeks, blood in your urine, nausea, chest pains, and sores in your mouth. There is a distinct possibility those are the symptoms of a chronic inflammatory disease called Lupus.

Lupus develops when your immune system produces antibodies that attack your body's own tissues. The theory is, Lupus is caused by an unknown virus that causes your immune system to develop antibodies in response to the viral attack. This causes a major malfunction of your immune system resulting in your body's own tissue being attacked.

There are several types of Lupus. The two major types are Systemic Lupus Erythematosus (SLE) and Discoid Lupus Erythematosus (DLE). There are also two less common forms of Lupus called Drug Induced Lupus and Neonatal Lupus.

Systemic Lupus (SLE)

When people refer to Lupus, they are generally referring to the Systemic type (SLE) because that is the type that effects the entire body. It can vary in intensity from mild to life threatening. Early symptoms often resemble the symptoms of arthritis such as swelling and pain in the joints. Additional symptoms such as chest pains, blood in the urine, ulcers, nausea, hair loss, and low grade fever has been reported. Approximately 33% of those who become afflicted with this disease will require medical attention.

In some of the more serious cases, even the brain, lungs, and heart can become affected. Early treatment can possibly prevent the central nervous system from becoming involved. If that were to happen, headaches, psychosis, serious depression, mania, seizures, and even stroke could become a distinct possibility. Being afflicted with Lupus makes a person prone to heart attack, infection, and kidney failure.

Discoid Lupus (DLE)

A less serious type of Lupus is called Discoid Lupus (DLE). This type of Lupus basically affects the skin with the traditional butterfly rash over the nose and cheeks. Lesions on the scalp and ears also appear, and last for an extended period of time, sometimes for years. The lesions will appear as small soft bumps, yellow in color, often leaving scars after they disappear. If the scars happen to be on the scalp, they often leave hairless patches in their wake. While Discoid Lupus is not life threatening, or even a threat to health, it can be seriously disfiguring.

Both types of Lupus have alternating periods of flare-ups and remission. Those who suffer from Discoid Lupus are highly susceptible to attacks if they are exposed to the sun's ultraviolet rays. Attacks can also be brought on by exposure to certain chemicals, drugs, or viral infections. If the case is drug induced, discontinuing the drug usually solves the problem.

A Holistic Approach To The Treatment Of Lupus

Numerous herbs have been studied for the treatment of Lupus. Several herbs like Reishi Mushroom, Cordyceps, and Nettles are of particular interest to those suffering from Lupus because of their ability to stimulate your immune system and to relieve pain.

It is advisable for persons afflicted with Lupus to avoid direct sunlight and to take protective measures if exposure is unavoidable. Protective measures in the form of sunscreen, wide-brimmed hats, and long sleeved garments that will adequately cover exposed skin is advisable.

Florescent lighting should be avoided at home and in the work place because exposure to this type of lighting can aggravate the symptoms of Lupus. If possible, it is advisable to remove all halogen and florescent lighting from the home and replace them with incandescent lighting.

Autoimmune diseases like Lupus can make a person more susceptible to infections, so avoiding large groups of people during the cold and flu seasons is advisable.

One should try to eat more eggs, garlic, and onions because they contain much needed sulfur for the repair and rebuilding of your bones, cartilage, and connective tissue.

Eating fresh pineapple on a regular basis allows Bromelain, an enzyme present in pineapple, to reduce inflammation. If you choose not to eat fresh pineapple, Bromelain supplements are available at your local supermarket or health food stores.

Try to avoid milk, dairy products, red meat (especially grain fed), citrus fruits, salt, tobacco, and anything containing sugar.

Mild cases of Lupus can be successfully treated with supplements that support y our immune system.

For more information on how to fine tune your immune system please refer to the following chapter.

A Parting Notation

I'm sure you have noticed, after reading this book, that you can prevent and even cure many of the ailments mentioned, and even some of those not mentioned, by simply keeping your immune system at peek efficiency. So in closing, this next chapter is appropriately devoted to your immune system, how it works, and how to improve it.

Your Immune System

Your immune system is your body's defense against all toxic invaders. Anything that attempts to enter your body with the intention of doing bodily harm is targeted and attacked with vigor. Let me clarify that statement. Attacked with vigor providing, you are a healthy person in excellent condition.

The most significant elements of your immune system are the Spleen, the Bone Marrow, and the Thymus Gland. Other significant players on this team are Enzymatic Proteins and the Lymphatic System with white blood cells and Lymphocytes which make up the backbone of your immune system.

Your healthy immune system is on guard 24/7 searching for antigens (proteins) that don't belong in your body. It can defend against a variety of invaders such as bacteria, viruses, parasites, and fungus. It can also recognize potential antigens such as insect venom, drugs, pollens, and chemicals. And as we all know, your immune system can recognize foreign tissue like transplanted organs. How many times have you heard on the news, "the organ transplant was a success, now there is a waiting period to see if the patient's body will reject the transplanted organ".

As mentioned earlier, your immune system functions at peak efficiency if you are a healthy person in excellent condition. Is your immune system functioning at peak efficiency ? There's a quick way to find out. Do you get chronic infections on a regular basis, do you get colds and the flu, or do you get nail fungus or respiratory allergies? If you answered yes to any of those questions then your immune system could probably use a tune-up.

So if your immune system is not functioning at peak efficiency, what is the reason ? There could be any number of reasons. Tops on the list are diet and nutrition. If your diet consists of fast foods, soft drinks, fried foods and sweet treats, then your immune system will suffer. If you use antibiotics on a regular basis, use drugs (over the counter, prescription, or illegal), if you smoke or live with a smoker, or if you consume more than two alcoholic drinks a day on a regular basis, your immune system will suffer.

Improving Your Immune System

Your immune system is your protector. It keeps you safe from all the potential ailments out there. Those ailments come in the form of diseases, virus, bacterial infections, too many to name on an individual basis. There are so many diseases and ailments out there waiting for just a little flaw in your immune systems defenses that it takes volumes of medical books to cover them all. At last count approximately 12,000.

And to make matters worse, there are new ailments developing on a regular basis. And, believe it or not, a well-tuned immune system can handle anything that comes it's way. The key phrase here is well-tuned. In order to keep your immune system well-tuned you will need to perform maintenance and preventive maintenance on a regular basis.

Let's take a look at preventative maintenance. Today's diet for our fast paced society consists of fast food, processed food, 21% sugar, and 38% fat which all suppress immune function. The saturated fats in pastries, fried foods, and grain fed beef are the main culprits.

Refined sugar is also a major immune suppressant. If a person were to consume a large candy bar at 8AM, that person's immune function would be vulnerable to attack until 1PM. The enemies of your immune system love sugar. During those five hours, sugar is destroying the ability of the white blood cells to kill germs, and the bad guys have a five hour window of opportunity.

Let's say "candy man", who had just eaten a candy bar, were to get into a crowded elevator and an infected person were to sneeze in his direction. You guessed it, "candy man" has just caught what "sneeze man" had. What if, later that morning, "candy man" picked up a telephone an infected person had just coughed on, now "candy man" is also infected. So in the last five hours while "candy man's" immune system was compromised, he has picked up a virus from the elevator and a bacterial infection from the office telephone. "Candy man" will be calling in sick tomorrow. If you must have a sweet snack, eat it at home before you go to bed, assuming no family members are sick.

The following list of supplements are key players on the immune system support team.

Vitamin A

If a Vitamin-A supplement were to be given to a malnourished child in a third world country, it could possibly save that child's life. If 25,000 international units of Beta-Carotene, a forerunner of the Vitamin-A supplement, were to be given to an adult every day, it could quite possibly help prevent Macular Degeneration (a major cause of blindness in people over the age of 50).

Needless to say, a Vitamin-A supplement could make a highly positive impact on your life. Without the proper amount of Vitamin-A, approximately 5000 International units, your body is open to the attack of a multitude of infections and diseases, even blindness. A Vitamin-A supplement can lower the risk of contracting many types of cancers and keep your immune system functioning at its peak. The ideal dosage of 5000 international units will also help guard against brittle bones, unhealthy skin, unhealthy gums, poor teeth, diarrhea, and respiratory infections.

With all these great things Vitamin-A supplements can offer, it might be a little tempting to double or even triple the dosage for even better results. Resist that temptation. Too much of a good thing is oftentimes a bad thing. Remember when you were a kid and your parents told you that eating too much candy would make you sick ? Did you believe them ? Nooo! Then the time came at a birthday party or a holiday event when you over indulged in some tasty sweets and you came to realize Mom and Dad were right. That same analogy holds true for Vitamin-A. The RDA is 5000 International units. Going over 5000 can potentially cause headaches, joint pain, weakness, blurred vision, and a multitude of other health issues. Moderation is the key word, don't be greedy.

Vitamin B-12

Cobalamin supplements (Vitamin B-12) is extremely important to the normal daily functions of a healthy body. It is instrumental in the production of red blood cells, plays a major role in the normal function of the nervous system, and helps to metabolize the body's fat and protein. The B-Vitamin family is often referred to as the brain vitamins. If that is the case, Vitamin B-12 would be classified as the head of the family because the lack of it can severely diminish a person's mental health. It is estimated that 15% of the people over age 65 are deficient in this important B-Vitamin.

As we get older we are prone to develop a condition called Atrophic Gastritis. This means there is a decrease in gastric acid and an increase of bacteria in the upper portion of the small intestine and the stomach. That combination seems to restrict the body's effort to take advantage of

Vitamin B-12's positive qualities. Taking additional Vitamin B-12 supplements should eliminate that problem. When shopping for Vitamin B-12 supplements look for the liquid form containing Methylcobalamin.

So what should you look for if you suspect a Vitamin B-12 deficiency ? If you or someone you love starts to show signs of neurological or psychological disturbances with no apparent physical cause, that person should be checked for a possible Vitamin deficiency. Actually, anyone over age 65 should be checked for a Vitamin B-12 deficiency on a regular basis (every year). A long term deficiency could cause serious problems. Take your B Vitamins also, not just B-12. A Vitamin B Complex capsule would be a good idea.

Vitamin C

Vitamin C (ascorbic acid) is known to prevent the common cold. It also protects the oral cavity, the stomach, the pancreas, and numerous other organs from cancer. Since Vitamin C is an antioxidant, it can delay or even prevent the formation of cataracts. This is how the whole process works. We know ultra violet light and oxidative stress in the lens of the eye are the major cause of cataract formation. We also know Vitamin C helps prevent the damage caused by oxidative stress.

If you happen to catch a cold, the common theory is to load up on Vitamin C. Everyone has heard that one. So is that fact for fiction ? That's a fact. Research has proven that high intake of this water soluble vitamin acts as a stimulant for some of our immune system's major defensive cells, stimulating them to move faster as they track down viruses and harmful bacteria. This action results in the prevention of a common cold or, at least a shortened duration of an existing cold.

People have been known to take extremely high doses of Vitamin C with no adverse effects. Others have experienced diarrhea. If you elect to take high doses, start slowly with 500 mg and work your way upwards. If you have a history of kidney stones, avoid high doses of this vitamin. Do you suffer from chronic constipation ? If so, try increasing your dosage of Vitamin C until your bowel movements become regular. That would be the perfect way to rid your body of those harmful toxic wastes while adding quality antioxidant coverage. A win-win situation.

Vitamin D

Vitamin D is known as the sunshine vitamin because if you spend 15 to 20 minutes in the sun you will get your daily requirements of the vitamin. Vitamin D is a major player in our unending quest for natural health excellence, and combined with Calcium and Phosphorus, it enables us to have strong bones. I shudder to think where we would be without a strong superstructure.

As we age our bodies produce less Vitamin D and the use of sunscreen prevents the sun's rays from producing Vitamin

D. And as we age our bodies are not as efficient at converting Vitamin D into the hormone needed to supply Calcium to our bones. If you are avoiding direct sunlight, not a bad idea, and you do not eat Vitamin D rich foods, you may not be getting enough Vitamin D into your system. Foods rich in Vitamin D are low or no fat dairy products, and fatty fish like salmon, mackerel, sardines, and tuna.

If you elect to take Vitamin D supplements, the RDA is 400 IU. During the winter months however, women need 500 IU to prevent bone loss.

So here is some good advice for women. Take a Vitamin D3 supplement of 400 IU or higher in the summer and winter. And compliment that with Chelated Calcium plus Magnesium supplements to keep your bones strong. Another strong case for taking supplements and vitamins.

Vitamin E

Vitamin E came onto the scene 65 years ago and we are still learning new things about these types of remarkable Antioxidants. Countless studies have proven that people who take Vitamin E on a regular basis are less likely to become afflicted with heart disease than those who do not take the vitamin.

In one study involving tens of thousands of registered female nurses and an equal amount of male medical professionals, it was found that those who consumed a minimum of 100 IU of Vitamin E a day had a 40% reduced risk of contracting heart disease. And to my knowledge, you will be hard pressed to find a Vitamin E supplement for less than 400 IU. And it seems as if many forward thinking cardiologists are starting to prescribe Vitamin E for their heart patients.

As we age our body functions begin to slow down and that is when age related problems start to show up. One of the major reasons these age related problems occur is because your immune system is one of those body functions that starts to slow down. This results in infections finding their way in, the common cold seems to last longer than it did when you were younger, and other ailments start to show up.

The flu, which was a minor inconvenience during your younger days, can be life threatening for an older person. Vitamin E has the ability to improve your immune function regardless of your age. The recommended daily allowance (RDA) for vitamin E is 400 IU daily. If you are over age 40, use the dry version because it is absorbed better.

Coenzyme Q10 (Co-Q10)

An enzyme is a protein in living cells that brings on a chemical change in the cells. A coenzyme works with an enzyme to produce a specific reaction. Coenzyme-Q10, commonly known as Co-Q10, is found in virtually every cell in the body and is instrumental in initiating the process that provides the cells with their energy. Unfortunately, as we get older our level of Co-Q10 declines. However, we can raise that level with exercise, eating healthy, and taking supplements. Since the mid-1970s, Co-Q10 has been used by the Japanese to treat heart disease and the aging process. A supplement that delays the aging process, how cool is that?

If you are a heart patient with angina pain and feeling tired all the time, try taking some Co-Q10. There is a good chance your angina pain will go away and your energy level will soar. Research has proven that consuming Co-Q10 supplements can also lower blood pressure, thus reducing the chances of having a stroke or a heart attack.

It's common knowledge that Free Radicals, unstable oxygen molecules that damage healthy cells, are the proverbial bad guys of our cellular system. And we also know that Antioxidants are the mortal enemy of Free Radicals. Co-Q10 is an Antioxidant, the Free Radical's worst enemy. The thought of Co-Q10s roaming around out there makes Free Radicals wake up screaming and the rest of us sleep like a baby.

If you choose to take Co-Q10 supplements take 100 mg with Ubiquinol.

Garlic

Garlic supplements have gone by many names like the stinking rose and Russian Penicillin, to name just a few. It has been used for more than 4000 years as an herbal medication. It is a natural Antibiotic and proved its worth during World War II when Penicillin was in short supply. It was used to fight the infections of wounded soldiers on the battlefield. Garlic is also a valuable tool in the fight against heart disease and blood clots which can cause heart attack and stroke.

Since it has been around for such a long time, a lot of research has been done on this very popular herb. The following are some of the results of that research.

1. Garlic has the unique ability to reduce the growth of Prostate Cancer cells.
2. Aged garlic (not fresh) reduces the body's production of Prostate-Specific Antigen (PSA) which can cause prostate cancer cells to grow.
3. Studies have shown that people who eat a lot of garlic have fewer colon and stomach cancers.
4. Garlic has been proven to boost immunity and reduce high blood sugar levels.
5. It relieves Asthma symptoms, keeping individual cells healthy and strong.
6. It contains numerous Sulfur compounds which help blood circulation, thus preventing platelets from sticking together to form clots.
7. Fresh organic or supplemental Garlic can prevent Cancer.
8. Garlic contains compounds that assist in preventing Nitrites from forming. Nitrites are a common substance found in foods like bacon and other cured

meats. Nitrites transform into Nitrosamines which are harmful compounds that can trigger Cancerous metabolic changes in our body's cells.

If you are a proponent of herbal health, it would make good sense to add this versatile herb to your repertoire.

Resveratrol

A while back, the wine drinking community was seriously excited about some news they had just heard. Scientists had confirmed it, drinking red wine has numerous health benefits such as reducing the risk of heart disease and inhibiting the formation of cancerous tumors.

Finally, an alcoholic drink that's good for you. Well, kinda good. Let's get one thing straight, it's not the alcohol that makes it good. It's actually the ingredients from the grape skin that presents the health benefits. The alcohol just comes along for the ride. So basically you have a good news bad news situation which in reality takes us back to square one. The researchers were painfully aware of that fact so they continued their research adding another team from a major university.

The new team discovered that all-important ingredient in the grape skin, resveratrol. Additional research discovered resveratrol could possibly prevent heart disease in two significant ways. First, it prevents the formation of blood clots, the major culprit in the proliferation of heart attack and stroke. Second, it is a major contributor to the metabolism of cholesterol which may prevent the formation of artery clogging plaque.

Is that not some seriously good news ? Well there's more. Resveratrol is a major player in the fight against cancer. In studies of human leukemia cells, resveratrol retarded the formation of abnormal cells and was able to turn malignant cells back to normal.

Until now, the only way you could reap the benefits of resveratrol was to drink red wine, lots of red wine. Now resveratrol is available in supplemental form. You would have to drink gallons of red wine to obtain an equal amount of resveratrol contained in one capsule.

Olive Leaf Extract

We've been eating olives and cooking with olive oil for thousands of years. But what about olive leaf extract, what is that ? It's an herbal supplement used to treat a multitude of ailments that has recently captured the attention of the world's most talented researchers. Most of those researchers have been from Europe but lately some prominent researchers from the United States have begun their own research programs.

This is what they found. The olive leaf contains a biologically energized compound that has significant antibacterial and antiviral properties. It interferes with the growth of bacteria and viruses while stimulating the activity of cells in the immune system that fight infection.

Olive leaf extract has successfully treated patients with chronic viral and bacterial infections. Many of those same patients had been previously treated, unsuccessfully, with numerous sessions of antibiotics. According to documented research, olive leaf extract is effective against a multitude of ailments including the herpes virus, bladder infections, bacterial infections, fungal infections, colds and the flu, shingles, chronic fatigue, HIV, pneumonia, blood poison, ear infections, urinary tract infections, and surgical infections (which seem to be happening a lot lately).

Actually, if you or someone you love are scheduled for a surgical procedure, it would be a good idea to start an olive leaf extract program well before and well after the procedure. An even better idea would be to make an olive leaf extract program part of your every-day activity because it seems as if this would be a very valuable supplement to have on your side.

Numerous highly respectable research labs have tested olive leaf extract and collectively they have discovered at least 120 illnesses to be positively effected by it. They have also discovered olive leaf extract kills 56 pathogens (disease producing organisms).

A Few Facts For You To Ponder

Mainstream medicine is big business and we all know the ultimate goal of any successful business is to have repeat customers (they want that to be you). Pharmaceuticals are developed to treat ailments that already exist, not to prevent ailments. Some of their side effects are often worse than the ailments they are trying to treat. If you have any doubts, just pay close attention to some of their TV commercials.

Numerous herbs, vitamins, and minerals are capable of preventing ailments, and most have little or no side effects. The choice is yours. As the intelligent and practical person I believe you are, I have a pretty good idea what your choice will be.

Congratulations.

Look for future books by Sauciron on Holistic Health. To stay informed on all updates, go to VitaminAndHerbalHealth. com and sign up for information on future publications by Sauciron.

www.ingramcontent.com/pod-product-compliance
Lightning Source LLC
Chambersburg PA
CBHW070750290526
45795CB00002B/547